A Journal for Healing

Cathy N. Moore, Ph.D.

and

Robin Freeman Bernstein, M.A.

A Main Street Book

Doubleday

New York London Toronto Sydney Auckland

A Journal for Healing

Writing Through Pain and Illness

A MAIN STREET BOOK
PUBLISHED BY DOUBLEDAY
a division of Bantam Doubleday Dell Publishing Group, Inc.
1540 Broadway, New York, New York 10036

MAIN STREET BOOKS, DOUBLEDAY, and the portrayal of a building with a tree are trademarks of Doubleday, a division of Bantam Doubleday Dell Publishing Group, Inc.

Book design by Maria Carella
Border decoration by Joanna Roy

The authors gratefully acknowledge permission to reprint from the following work:
Jaffe, Hirshel, and Poller, H. Leonard, eds. *Gates of Healing*. New York: Central Conference of American Rabbis, 1988. Used by permission.

ISBN 0-385-48184-5

Printed in the United States of America

May 1996

1 3 5 7 9 10 8 6 4 2

First Edition

To my father, Tom Moore, and
my brother, Alan Moore

Love, Cathy

To my father, Leonard Freeman;
my special colleague and friend, Bonnie Sturner Ph.D.; and
my beloved friend and teacher, Bob Gibson

Love, Robin

and

To all the courageous people who
are now holding this book

Love, Cathy and Robin

Contents

3. Sample Journal Entries and Letters

INTRODUCTION FROM CATHY AND ROBIN

Dear Friend,

Welcome. You are holding *A Journal for Healing* because you have been given a diagnosis or are living with an illness. We are truly aware of the tremendous impact and change this brings to your life. We hope journaling will bring much peace and companionship to you as you travel your path. Although it may feel as if you have never had such an experience before or felt these feelings, it's quite possible you have.

Before you were born, you lived within your mother's womb. It was safe, warm, quiet, and peaceful. You were comfortable, and everything you needed was provided. For nine months your world was familiar and undisturbed.

Then, boom! The world as you once knew it began suddenly to change. You were jolted, moved around by some unknown force and pushed into an entirely new world. You were greeted with a slap on the bottom, bright lights, a change in temperature, and clothing. Everything was different. "Where am I and what's going on?"—these were your thoughts as you cried and looked around.

Thankfully, you were placed in arms that loved and cared for you. Feeling this, you calmed down. But inwardly you were unsure, confused, scared and uncomfortable. It would take you a while to become familiar with your new world.

Receiving a diagnosis from a doctor is much like being born. You leave a familiar world and enter into a new, unfamiliar and often scary one. Instead of the shock of noise, bright lights, and clothing, you may find yourself experiencing the shock of a diagnosis, a foreign language of medical terminology, and uncertainty. Your life as you have lived it begins to change, sometimes at a very rapid pace.

It is for this reason we have written *A Journal for Healing*. It is for you—the individual whose life has once again suddenly changed and begun anew.

A Journal for Healing understands what you are experiencing, possibly even before you do. It will be your companion, and through your journal entries and the writing of letters to family, friends, and children will give you strength, comfort, and a sense of control. In your hands you hold a source of help as you travel through this challenging—and often enlightening—time in your life.

We created this journal after many years of having guided and cared for family, friends, and clients living with illness. Over and over again, the combination of a personal journal and the intimacy of letter writing empowered them with inner strength, clarity, resolve, understanding, and peace. Then, toward the end of our writing this book, Cathy Moore was diagnosed with breast cancer. On a daily basis she now faces decisions related to treatment, physical changes, lifestyle changes, and the emotional issues that accompany living with this illness. Through our research and our experience with clients, family, and friends—and now, Cathy's challenge—we have had the opportunity to see and hear closely the many benefits our form of guided journal and letter writing brings. Benefits described to us include the following:

- "The paper does not judge me or try to change me. It listens unconditionally, and on each page I can let go of the old and have a fresh start."
- "Writing takes me out of the difficult world around me, and while I'm writing I can focus on me and me alone."
- "My journal is a place where I can say anything I want and anything I feel."
- "Writing helps me get in touch with my feelings—the feelings I'm unable to talk about. Once I write about my feelings, it's easier for me to talk about them."
- "Writing is like emptying out a closet that is filled to the brim: I don't like doing it, but it feels so good when it's done."

- "Letter writing lets me practice what I want to say to my family and friends. Sometimes I just give them the letters I wrote."
- "Sometimes I'm so overwhelmed inside, writing helps calm me down."
- "When I'm with my journal, I don't have to put on a brave front. I can be anxious, scared, angry, worried—whatever, I can just be me."
- "I wasn't allowed to express my feelings and emotions when I was a child, so I kept them bottled up inside. Seeing the topics at the top of the page helps me to face my feelings. Writing lets me release them and prevents me from denying I'm ill, and allows me to fight for my life. Writing is a rededication to myself and healing."
- "When I'm finished writing, I can leave my fears and concerns inside my journal and letters. I can take a break. They will be there if I wish to return to them."
- "My journal is there for me twenty-four hours a day. This is very comforting."

We now wish to extend this experience to you.

Part One of the book is your personal journal. We have provided topics that come from many sources, such as individuals who are living with a diagnosis and an illness; medical literature; mind-body-spirit research and documentaries. Topics include: "Today I became a patient . . ."; "I am courageous . . ."; "The middle of the night is a difficult time for me—there is so much internal chatter in my head when it is quiet. Let me write it out . . ." It is our hope that through the journaling process you will be able to face and accept your diagnosis/illness mentally, emotionally, and physically rather than letting the diagnosis/illness control you, your life, and your thoughts.

Part Two of the book is devoted to the writing of letters. When given a diagnosis or living with an illness, you'll find the writing of letters can help you stay connected to important people around you. Letters are a way to express your innermost feelings, thoughts, concerns, wishes, and hopes. Letter writing gives the writer emotional freedom—the release of a secret, the sharing of a difficult feeling, or even simply letting another person know how special and loved he or she is. This gives the writer inner strength and peace of mind. As Alexandra Stoddard says in her book *Gift of a Letter*, "A personal letter can be one of the most intimate and touching of human expressions, one to another. A letter is a gift signature of you."

Accompanying you on your journey of journal and letter writing will be sample journal entries and letters from others who have been given a diagnosis or have been living with an illness for some time now. They write about their many different feelings and experiences. These writings, shown in Part Three, are there to serve as a guide and touchstone for you as you begin this process.

Once again, welcome. May the writing in your journal and the writing of letters bring you understanding, clarity, acceptance, strength, comfort, and healing.

With respect and admiration,

Cathy and Robin

1

My Journal

HOW TO USE THIS JOURNAL

Dear Friend,

Welcome to the journal-writing part of this book. Here, you can write about feelings and experiences that can be hard to understand when you are first diagnosed and thus entering an unfamiliar world. In our work as therapists we have learned that for many people, journal writing can provide great insight, comfort, and healing. An important goal of the journal is to help you become closely connected with yourself, and you will find that this greater self-awareness enhances your relationships with those around you. There are three sections within your journal. They include: "After the Diagnosis—My Feelings," "Living with the Illness—My Feelings," and "Notes to Myself . . ."

We realize those who choose to enter the writing process will be at different and unique places in relation to their illness and the effect it is having on their emotional and physical well-being. Take your time and read through *A Journal for Healing*. Become familiar with the chapters. Then start writing at any place that relates to where you are.

When writing this book, we were also aware that many of you may be seasoned journal writers and will need very little guidance on how to use this section of the book. But some of you may be writing in a journal for the first time, and beginning one can be an awkward process. Our clients often asked the questions: "What do I write about?"; "I see the blank page and I don't know where to begin. How do I get started?"; "Do I need to fill the entire page?" So we became their guides, suggesting topics for them. Their hesitancy, confusion, and insecurity disappeared when they were given this guidance. We hope these topics will do the same for you.

The first two sections of your journal deal with your feelings. At the top of each page you will find a space to fill in the date and a suggested journal topic. Many of the topics will make you feel as if you'd written them yourself; others may not relate to you. If this happens, move on to a topic that reflects how you feel at the moment. You may choose to write in the suggested order of the topics, or you can skip around and go in your own order. There are no "have-to"s. If topics we suggest don't inspire you, feel free to write your own journal entries on the blank pages provided. You may even choose to meditate or reflect on a topic inwardly without writing a word. Your journal and the topics provided can serve as a catalyst. Where you go from there is totally in your control and is up to you.

The last section of "My Journal" is called "Notes to Myself . . ." It is organized in a different way from the first two sections. "Notes to Myself . . ." is devoted to specific areas that concern the individual with an illness, such as "Doctor/Treatment," "Finances," "Body Changes," and "My Pleasures/Enjoyments." We realize some of the topics listed within these areas may apply to you and many may not. Therefore, instead of devoting a whole journal page to each topic, we've listed them together. If a topic in one of these areas connects with you, turn to one of the blank pages that follow. Record the date, enter the topic of your choice in the space provided, and begin writing.

Your journal is there for you twenty-four hours a day. As you turn to it more and more, you will gain understanding about what you're going through and develop the inner strength to carry on.

Cathy and Robin

After the Diagnosis—My Feelings

When fate knocks you flat on your back,
remember she leaves you looking up.
—Anonymous

Date:

TOPIC: *I've just received the diagnosis and I'm in shock . . .*

Date:

TOPIC: *Why me? . . .*

Date:

TOPIC: *I'm going to ask for a second opinion . . .*

Date: ______________________________

TOPIC: *I went to the bookstore and bought a wonderful book. It's called ______________________. It helps me by . . .*

Knowledge is the food of the soul.

—PLATO

Date: ______________________

TOPIC: *I bought all these great books to help me understand what's going on inside my body and they are still in the trunk of my car . . .*

Date: ______

TOPIC: *I'm doing research so I can learn about the diagnosis. I want to participate in my own treatment and recovery . . .*

Take up, read! Take up, read!
—ST. AUGUSTINE

Date: ______________________

TOPIC: *I bought this journal and I can't even write in it yet . . .*

We can do anything we want to do
if we stick to it long enough.
—HELEN KELLER

Date:

TOPIC: *How will I tell my children? . . .*

Date: ______________________________

TOPIC: *How will I tell my parents . . .*

Date: ______________________

TOPIC: *Today I became a patient . . .*

The beginning is the most important part of the work.
—PLATO

Date: ______

TOPIC: *I am apprehensive about what comes next . . .*

Faith is the substance of things hoped for,
the evidence of things not seen.
—HEBREWS 11:1

Date:

TOPIC: *I was told I need surgery . . .*

Date:

TOPIC: *My mind is reeling/racing out of control . . .*

Date: ______

TOPIC: *I'm taking it one step at a time . . .*

Date: ____________________

TOPIC: *I want to live . . .*

Your heaviest artillery (in sickness) will be your will to live. Keep that big gun going.
—NORMAN COUSINS

Date: ____________________

TOPIC: *I'm willing to change . . .*

Date:

TOPIC: *Friends and family have been so supportive. What has truly touched me is . . .*

Date:

TOPIC: *I'm not going to let statistics scare me or control my thoughts . . .*

The present is our own.
—THOMAS LOVE PEACOCK

Date: ____________________

TOPIC: *When night time comes and the house is quiet, I find . . .*

Date: ______________________

TOPIC: *I'm feeling so vulnerable . . .*

Date:

TOPIC: *Sometimes I feel this disease is my fault, even though I am told it is not . . .*

Date: ______

TOPIC: *What is the message, the teaching, of this disease/illness for me and my own life today?* . . .

Date: ______________________

TOPIC: *I need to work because it gives me a break from thinking about the illness . . .*

Date: ______________________

TOPIC: *I'm going to the hospital . . .*

Date: ___

TOPIC: *Today I need lots of love, especially from myself . . .*

Self-love . . . is not so vile a sin
as self-neglecting.
—WILLIAM SHAKESPEARE

Date:

TOPIC: *I am in physical pain. What is the message the pain is giving me? . . .*

Date:

TOPIC: *I'm afraid I'm not going to heal . . .*

Date:

TOPIC: *I like being touched and hugged. It feels . . .*

Date: ______________________

TOPIC: *I've decided to see a mental health professional/therapist. I'm feeling . . .*

Date: ______________________

TOPIC: *Notes about being in therapy . . .*

Date:

TOPIC: *When I'm scared, I fear that the diagnosis is a very premature death sentence . . .*

Date: ______

TOPIC: *I've decided to join a support group. I'm feeling . . .*

Date: ______

TOPIC: *Notes about being in a support group . . .*

Date: ______________________

TOPIC: *Today I told* ______________ *about the diagnosis . . .*

Date: ______________________________

TOPIC: *I am free to experience whatever I feel today. I will not judge my feelings . . .*

Live in this moment and live in eternity.
—JOHANN WOLFGANG VON GOETHE

Date:

TOPIC: *Today I had a good cry . . .*

For this relief much thanks.
—WILLIAM SHAKESPEARE

Date: ______________________

TOPIC: *Today I am down in the dumps. I don't want to get dressed, open the shades, or talk with anyone. For today I will be free to experience being down in the dumps . . .*

To do nothing is sometimes a good remedy.
—HIPPOCRATES

Date: ______

TOPIC: *I feel myself pulling away from everybody . . .*

Do what you can, with what you have,
with where you are.
—THEODORE ROOSEVELT

Date: ______________________

TOPIC: *I'm so angry . . .*

Date: ____________________

TOPIC: *Since the diagnosis, I am facing my own mortality. I'm feeling . . .*

Date: ______

T O P I C : *I'm taking a break today from dealing with the illness. I'm feeling . . .*

Date: ______________________

TOPIC: *What I love about my life is . . .*

Date: ______________________

TOPIC: *What I love about myself is . . .*

Date: ___

TOPIC: *Dreams . . . Thoughts . . . Poems . . .*

Date:

TOPIC: *Dreams . . . Thoughts . . . Poems . . .*

Date:

TOPIC: *Dreams . . . Thoughts . . . Poems . . .*

Living with the Illness— My Feelings

In the midst of winter, I finally learned that there was
in me an invincible summer.
—Albert Camus

Date: ______________________

T O P I C : *I have a newly deepened appreciation for life . . .*

Finish every day and be done with it. You have done what you could. Some blunders and absurdities no doubt crept in; forget them as soon as you can. Tomorrow is a new day; begin it well and serenely and with too high a spirit to be cumbered with your old nonsense. This day is all that is good and fair. It is dear, with its hopes and invitations, to waste a moment on yesterdays.

—RALPH WALDO EMERSON

Date: ____________________

TOPIC: *Having someone to listen to me helps so much . . .*

Date: ______________________

TOPIC: *Even though I'm feeling uncomfortable today (physically or mentally), I'm not going to let this discomfort ruin my day . . .*

Date: __________

TOPIC: *My sense of humor . . .*

Date: ____________________

TOPIC: *Friends/family are opposed to the form of treatment I've chosen. This leaves me feeling . . .*

Date: ______________________

TOPIC: *Whenever I feel any new physical discomfort, I wonder if it's the disease progressing. When this happens, I feel . . .*

Date: ______________________

TOPIC: *I'm having trouble sleeping . . .*

Date: ______________________________

TOPIC: *I'm suffering right now—and I wonder how much more suffering I can endure . . .*

When pain and fatigue are my companions,
Let there be room in my heart for strength.
When days and nights are filled with darkness,
Let the light of courage find its place.
Help me to endure the suffering and dissolve
the fear. Renew within me the calm spirit of
trust and peace.

—FROM *GATES OF HEALING*

Date: ____________________

TOPIC: *If it weren't for the children (husband, friends, lover), I'd be tempted to . . .*

Date: ______________________________

TOPIC: *I'm feeling angry (or ________________) about plans I made for my life and for my future. The illness threatens the possibility of their happening . . .*

Date: ______________________________

TOPIC: *I can't find the words to express the anger I'm feeling. Let me draw the anger . . .*

Date:

TOPIC: *I'm scared . . .*

Date: ______________________________

TOPIC: *I can't find the words to express the fear I'm feeling. Let me draw the fear . . .*

Date: ______________________

TOPIC: *What gives me strength is . . . (greater clarity and understanding, appreciation of time, the ability to live in the moment . . .)*

Date:

TOPIC: *Sometimes I still feel this disease is my fault, even though I now know it is not . . .*

Date: ______________________

TOPIC: *I'm mourning the loss of my life as I once knew it so I can move on to my life as it is today . . .*

Date: ______

T O P I C : *I wonder if I can recover physically . . .*

Date:

TOPIC: *I find myself making up pictures in my mind of events that aren't even happening . . .*

Date: ______________________

TOPIC: *I find myself taking in each moment and savoring it . . .*

Date: ________________________________

TOPIC: *I'm taking it one step at a time . . .*

I never think of the future.
It comes soon enough.
—ALBERT EINSTEIN

Date: ______

TOPIC: *Today I'm feeling lonely . . .*

Date: ______________________________

T O P I C : *Memories that give me strength during this difficult time . . .*

Date: ____

TOPIC: *Being interested in others helps me not to focus so much on myself. It helps because . . .*

Date: ______

TOPIC: *Wonderful opportunities to heal are all around me . . .*

Ask, and it shall be given you; seek, and ye shall find; knock, and it shall be opened unto you.
—MATTHEW 7:7

Date: ______________________

TOPIC: *I wish people would stop asking me how I feel or treating me like a victim . . .*

Date: ______________________

TOPIC: *It feels so good when other people talk with me about how they're doing since I was given this diagnosis . . .*

Date: ______

TOPIC: *While I was sitting and waiting for treatment, a woman/man shared a story that gave him/her the strength to go on. I always want to remember those words of wisdom and that story of hope . . .*

Date: ______________________________

TOPIC: *Today I need lots of love, especially from myself . . .*

Self-love is the instrument of our preservation.
—VOLTAIRE

Date:

TOPIC: *I've decided to write my will. I feel . . .*

Date: ______________________________

TOPIC: *I feel better that* ____________________ *is no longer a secret . . .*

Date: ______________________________

TOPIC: *I am limited by the illness. I'm feeling . . .*

Date: ______

TOPIC: *I pray for . . .*

Date: ______________________________

TOPIC: *Let me clear away the resentments I have toward people and events in my life. Holding on to them places an added burden . . .*

To be wronged is nothing unless you continue to remember it.

—CONFUCIUS

Date: ______________________

TOPIC: *My children feel . . .*

Date:

TOPIC: *My partner/spouse doesn't understand . . .*

Date: ______________________

T O P I C : *It's back to the hospital . . .*

God, I'm tired of this whole hospital experience! In fact, I'm fed up with it. I'm bored. The days and nights just drag by. The routine of sleeping and eating, temperature and blood pressure taking, is about to get me down. The noise in the hallway bothers me, too. Not much seems to be happening. I want to go home! You don't have to tell me—I know what my problem is. I need to be more patient. I can't expect to get well overnight. Healing takes time. Strength doesn't return with the snap of my fingers. So, make me aware that if I can endure a little more and a little longer, these experiences will be behind me. And when I look back on them, they won't seem so frustrating as they do right now. Amen.

—FROM *GATES OF HEALING*

Date:

TOPIC: *I am courageous . . .*

Date: ______________________________

TOPIC: *Today I had a good cry . . .*

We must always change, renew, rejuvenate ourselves; otherwise we harden.
—JOHANN WOLFGANG VON GOETHE

Date: ______

TOPIC: *The physical pain leaves me feeling depressed . . .*

Date: ______

TOPIC: *Life has been difficult and filled with pain. Let me write about ways to re-create my life in order to once again give it new meaning and purpose . . .*

Date:

TOPIC: *I'm learning to move into and through the pain . . .*

Date: ______________________________

TOPIC: *I am free to experience whatever I feel today. I will not judge my feelings . . .*

Date: ______________________________

TOPIC: *Being around other people with the same illness is good for me . . .*

Date: ______________________________

T O P I C : *I can't find the words to express the faith I'm feeling. Let me draw faith . . .*

Date: ______

T O P I C : *I like being touched. It feels so good . . .*

Date: ______________________

TOPIC: *Sleep is healing . . .*

May it be Your will that I lie down in peace and rise up in peace. Let not my thoughts, my dreams, or my daydreams disturb me. Watch over my family and those I love. Grant me a night of rest. Let the healing processes that You have placed in my body go about their work. May I awaken in the morning, refreshed and renewed to face a new tomorrow.

—FROM *GATES OF HEALING*

Date:

TOPIC: *Just what is my purpose to go on living? . . .*

The important thing is not to stop questioning.
—ALBERT EINSTEIN

Date: ______________________________

TOPIC: *Swallowing emotions (anger, guilt, fear, insecurity . . .) or pretending they are not there is like poison to me. Let me write out the emotions . . .*

Date: ______________________

TOPIC: *My life revolves around my treatment and medication schedules. I'm feeling . . .*

Date: ______

TOPIC: *I feel people don't understand what I'm going through, and that leaves me feeling distant from them . . .*

Date:

TOPIC: *I am sick of feeling sick all the time . . .*

Date: ______________________________

TOPIC: *I've decided to see a mental health professional . . .*

Date: ______________________

T O P I C : *These are my notes about being in therapy . . .*

Date: ______________________________

TOPIC: *I'm going to work even though I feel far from 100 percent. My feelings about working are . . .*

Date: ______________________

TOPIC: *I feel I have to appear brave and cheerful as much as possible, because if I don't I'm afraid what I'm really feeling will scare people away . . .*

Date: ______________________

T O P I C : *I want to write down thoughts and feelings I have never told anyone before, even myself . . .*

Date:

TOPIC: *There is a part of me that likes being sick. Let me write out the benefits . . .*

Date: ______________________

TOPIC: *The middle of the night is a difficult time for me—there is so much internal chatter in my head when it is quiet. Let me write it out . . .*

Date: ______________________________

TOPIC: *I'm tired of living with the disease—it's a weight on my shoulders . . .*

Date: ________________

TOPIC: *I'm not handling the illness as well as I did in the beginning . . .*

Date: ______________________________

TOPIC: *Today was a special day because I . . .*

Date: ______________________

TOPIC: *I'm nervous that I won't be able to provide for my family . . .*

Date:

TOPIC: *I'm isolating myself from others . . .*

Date:

TOPIC: *I've decided to join a support group . . .*

Date: ______________________________

TOPIC: *These are my thoughts about being in a support group . . .*

Date: ____

TOPIC: *I'm scared to let my group really know me—my vulnerability, fears, mistakes, anger, sadness . . .*

You gain strength, courage, and confidence by every experience in which you really stop to look fear in the face. You are able to say to yourself, "I lived through this hour. I can take the next thing that comes along." You must do the thing you cannot do.

—ELEANOR ROOSEVELT

Date:

TOPIC: *I'm so proud of myself . . .*

Date:

TOPIC: *I'm in physical pain. What is the message the pain is giving me? . . .*

Date: __________

TOPIC: *I'm in emotional pain. What is the message the pain is giving me? . . .*

Date: ______________________________

TOPIC: *I respect and value myself and find that I am now taking care of myself in new and different ways . . .*

Date: ______

TOPIC: *Living with the illness has led me on a spiritual journey . . .*

Date: ______________________

TOPIC: *I'm accepting the changes in my body and in my life . . .*

God, give us grace to accept with serenity the things that cannot be changed, courage to change the things which should be changed, and the wisdom to distinguish the one from the other.

—REINHOLD NIEBUHR

Date: ______________________________

TOPIC: *The physical pain is under control . . .*

Date: ____________________

TOPIC: *I feel I can beat this illness—the possibility exists . . .*

Date: ________________________________

TOPIC: *I receive so much through writing. Writing is valuable because . . .*

Date:

TOPIC: *I'm scared I won't always be able to live on my own . . .*

Date:

TOPIC: *I have a live-in caregiver . . .*

Have you longed and struggled to be independent? Being independent is as impossible as the heart being independent of the rest of the body. Do like the heart . . . be dependent on others, but make a contribution to life.

—RHONDELL

Date: ______________________________

TOPIC: *I just realized I got through the day/night without thinking about the illness . . .*

It is a part of the cure to wish to be cured.
—SENECA

Date: ____________________

TOPIC: *I now do my best to live each day to the fullest . . .*

Date: ______________________

T O P I C : *I'm embarrassed about . . .*

Date: ____________________

TOPIC: *I am free to experience all feelings—pain, happiness, discomfort, love—because I know each feeling teaches me something and tells me I am alive . . .*

Date: ______________________________

TOPIC: *Getting through the day is easier now. I'm able to focus on living rather than the illness . . .*

May you live all the days of your life.
—JONATHAN SWIFT

Date: ______

TOPIC: *I'm so happy I've been able to . . .*

Date: ____________________

TOPIC: *If I stay in the present, I am fine. If I let my mind travel into the past or the future, I become anxious and worry. Inner peace is right here—now . . .*

The best thing about the future
is that it comes one day at a time.
—ABRAHAM LINCOLN

Date: ______________________________

TOPIC: *I'm healing . . .*

Healing does not necessarily mean to become physically well or to be able to get up and walk around again. Rather, it means achieving a balance between the physical, emotional, intellectual, and spiritual dimensions.

—ELISABETH KUBLER-ROSS

Date: ____

TOPIC: *I'm afraid I'm not going to heal . . .*

Date: ______________________________

TOPIC: *I know I'm healing emotionally and physically because I can look at the scar(s) on my body without getting upset . . .*

Date: ______________________________

TOPIC: *I am a survivor . . .*

Date:

TOPIC: *Dreams . . . Thoughts . . . Poems . . .*

Date:

TOPIC: *Dreams . . . Thoughts . . . Poems . . .*

Date:

TOPIC: *Dreams . . . Thoughts . . . Poems . . .*

Notes to Myself . . .

What lies behind us and what lies before us are tiny matters compared to what lies within us.

—Ralph Waldo Emerson

DOCTOR/TREATMENT

The patient must combat the disease
along with the physician.
—HIPPOCRATES

- In choosing doctors who will work with me, I look for . . .
- I'm keeping records of my phone conversations with my doctor . . .
- I'm going to ask my doctor to explain to me step by step what I may experience. This is what I've learned so far . . .
- I have an appointment with my doctor and I'm going to bring my tape recorder along. I'm doing this because . . .
- I replayed the tape from my doctor's visit. What I want to remember is . . . (questions, thoughts, feelings . . .)
- I'm finding I don't agree with my doctor . . .
- I'm going to try a new doctor . . .
- I have the power to choose the treatment that is best for me. The treatment plan I'm leaning toward is . . .
- I'm going to take my time making a decision for treatment, even if those around me are pressuring me to decide fast . . .
- I've decided to incorporate Eastern techniques into my treatment process . . . (acupuncture, herbs, meditation . . .)
- I'm more scared of the treatment than of the diagnosis . . .
- I've just begun a cycle of treatment . . .
- I have treatment today, and a way to nurture myself before is to . . .
- I have treatment today, and a way to nurture myself after is to . . .
- The side effects of treatment have been . . .
- Doctor's appointment today. I'm feeling . . .
- Part of my treatment is going to be to laugh and have fun. Today I . . .
- I've had a setback in treatment . . .

- I've just finished a cycle of treatment . . .
- It's in my best interest to communicate fully with my doctor what is going on inside my body so he/she can do the best for me. Sometimes I want to do this and sometimes I don't. Right now I feel . . .
- I have questions for my doctor and it's after hours. Even though I feel awkward calling, I'm going to ease my mind and call him/her. My questions are . . . His/her answers were . . .
- Time for a checkup. I'm feeling . . .
- Part of healing for me is being 100 percent responsible for my medication intake. I'm going to keep a log of my medication intake . . .
- My doctor has no bedside manner . . .
- I'm working with a hypnotherapist . . .
- I'm wearing a Medic Alert bracelet because . . .
- I'm in remission . . .
- I'm in recovery . . .

Date:

TOPIC:

Date:

TOPIC:

Date:

TOPIC:

Date:

TOPIC:

Date:

TOPIC:

THE HOSPITAL

- I want to have a friend or relative oversee my stay in the hospital. The person I'll ask . . .
- What I'll bring to the hospital . . .
- Before I go into the hospital, I'm bringing all the medications I take regularly or occasionally to my doctor to find out if it's okay to keep taking them, given the procedure I'm going into the hospital for. This is what she/he said . . .
- My doctors' phone numbers (surgeon, physician, anesthesiologist):

  Name ____________ Office ______________ Home ______________

  Name ____________ Office ______________ Home ______________

  Name ____________ Office ______________ Home ______________

- I'm having surgery . . .
- I'm going to keep the lines of communication open between me and my doctor(s). What I want to let him/her/them know is . . .
- The charge nurse's name is ____________________ . . .
- The physician in charge of me is ____________________ . . .
- Either I or my friend/relative will write down each meditation prescribed for me, paying special attention to:

  –The name

  –What it's for

  –What it looks like

  –When I am supposed to take it

- I'm going to ask my doctor if I'll be on a restricted diet or if I can have food brought in from the outside. She/he said . . .

- Thoughts on visitors . . .
- Thoughts about leaving the hospital . . .
- Books I'd like to read while I'm in the hospital . . .
- Memories of my hospital stay . . .

Date: __________

TOPIC: __________

Date:

TOPIC:

Date:

TOPIC:

Date:

TOPIC:

Date:

TOPIC:

LIFESTYLE CHANGES

- I'm slowly making changes that will enhance the quality of my life and that my doctor has recommended. I'm looking at the following areas:

  –Nutrition
  –Physical activity/exercise
  –Environment
  –Inner feelings

- Since making changes in this area, I notice I'm feeling . . .
- Sometimes it's hard to be consistent with these changes . . .
- I'm enjoying my new way of life . . .
- I now have someone living with me . . .
- I'm moving out of my home . . .
- I'm adjusting to the changes in my lifestyle. The one I want to write about is . . .

Date:

TOPIC:

Date:

TOPIC:

Date:

TOPIC:

Date:

TOPIC:

HOLIDAYS

- Birthday . . .
- Anniversary . . .
- Passover . . .
- Easter . . .
- Chanukah . . .
- Thanksgiving . . .
- Christmas . . .
- New Year's . . .
- And any others I wish to write about . . .

Date:

TOPIC:

Date:

TOPIC:

Date:

TOPIC:

Date: ______

TOPIC: ______

LOVEMAKING/SEXUALITY

- Since the illness, I've noticed a change in my sexual desires . . . (increase/decrease)
- Lovemaking scares me sometimes . . .
- I feel my partner is different with me when we make love now . . .
- Lovemaking is better than ever . . .
- Sometimes I like to be touched and sometimes I don't. Communicating this is . . . (easy, difficult, uncomfortable, scary . . .)
- When I'm naked with my partner . . .
- I'm concerned if lovemaking is still as wonderful for my partner . . .
- I'm worried about the changes in my body . . .

Date:

TOPIC:

Date:

TOPIC:

Date:

TOPIC:

Date:

TOPIC:

FINANCES

- How will I pay for this treatment? My plans . . .
- My feelings about my medical insurance . . .
- I'm shocked by how much my medication and treatment will cost . . .
- I'm glad I'm taking care of my finances . . .
- I'm doing my best to pay off all my bills so I can have a clean slate and clear all my debt . . .
- I wish I didn't even have to think about money at a time like this . . .
- Financial changes I'm making . . .
- People who are helping me financially . . .

Date:

TOPIC:

Date:

TOPIC:

Date:

TOPIC:

Date:

TOPIC:

BODY CHANGES

- I know my body is going to be changing. Here's how I feel today . . . (wondering, scared, apprehensive, accepting . . .)
- I'm sending a special good-bye and thank-you to the part of my body that will no longer be with me after tomorrow . . . (kidney, lung, breast, limb . . .)
- I look so different since the treatment began. I'm feeling uncomfortable . . . (being around friends, out in public . . .)
- I'm going to miss . . .
- I'm becoming more familiar with the changes in my body . . .
- I'm feeling thankful for what my body can do for me today . . .
- I'm learning how not to let the changes in my body control my moods. I'm doing this by . . .
- This is what is going on in my body now . . . (fatigue, strength, pain . . .)
- Even though I look different physically or my body is different, I realize I am still the same me inside . . . (courageous, witty, intelligent, warm . . .)
- My weight is changing, and here is how I feel . . .
- I'm feeling __________ about my body/physical appearance . . .
- Living with a prosthesis has been . . .
- When I'm naked, I feel . . .
- I'm angry about things I can't do right now/any longer . . .
- I feel as if my body has let me down . . .

Date:

TOPIC:

Date:

TOPIC:

Date: ________________

TOPIC:

Date:

TOPIC:

Date:

TOPIC:

MY PLEASURES/ENJOYMENTS

It is a happy talent to know how to play.
—RALPH WALDO EMERSON

- Music . . .
- Entertainment . . .
- Walks/hikes . . .
- Gardening . . .
- Sports . . .
- Friends/family/children/grandchildren . . .
- Pets . . .
- Meditating . . .
- Reading . . .
- Television/movies . . .
- Games . . .
- Art . . .
- Photography . . .
- Crafts . . .
- Cooking . . .
- Special memories . . .
- Other pleasures and enjoyments I have . . .

Date:

TOPIC:

Date:

TOPIC:

Date:

TOPIC:

Date:

TOPIC:

Date:

TOPIC:

2

My Letters

If we look at the path, we do not see the sky. We are earth people on a spiritual journey to the stars. Our quest, our earth walk, is to look within, to know who we are, to see that we are connected to all things, that there is no separation, only in the mind.

—Native American, source unknown

HOW TO USE THE LETTERS SECTION

Dear Friend,

The first part of this book was devoted to your journal, and to getting in touch with your thoughts, emotions, and experiences. The part you're now looking at, "My Letters," will help you stay connected with and communicate your feelings to those around you. Letter writing gives you the opportunity to express your inner thoughts, concerns, wishes, needs, and hopes. Some of these letters you will want to take from your journal and send to the person you're addressing. Others you may wish to keep to yourself. Sometimes the sole purpose of letter writing is to enable you to release frustrations, to vent uncomfortable feelings you don't feel safe communicating, or to clarify what your true feelings are. In each of these cases, we want you to know it is okay simply to keep the letters to yourself. Writing letters, whether you send them or not, is a healthy way to enhance your own inner strength and self-esteem.

We have divided "My Letters" into three sections: "Letters to My Partner/Spouse," "Letters to My Children," and "Letters to My Relatives and Friends." As with Part One, "My Journal," please know that you are welcome to begin any place you wish, skip around, or flip back and forth from section to section. Once again, it's up to you to choose the topics that reflect where you are in your life and your relationships.

As you look ahead, you will see that the design of the letters section is similar to that of the journal section. Date and suggested topic are at the top of many pages. There are also some pages with several suggested topics listed together. For example, under "Letters to My Children," the subsection "I Want to Share with You" begins with a list of ideas and experiences you may want to place within your letter. We realize you all will have different priorities of what you want to share; therefore, instead of devoting a whole page to each of these topics, we have listed them together. If a topic in one of these areas touches you and inspires a letter, turn to one of the blank pages that follow. On all the blank pages, you will see a space at the top to write in the date and the topic you have chosen. Of course, you may also create your own topics.

If by chance you need inspiration or direction, turn to Part Three, "Sample Journal Entries and Letters." There you will find guidance.

Cathy and Robin

Letters to My Partner/Spouse

Let there be truth between us two forevermore.
—Ralph Waldo Emerson

Date: ______________________________

TOPIC: *We've all been given a real challenge . . .*

Sorrow and silence are strong,
and patient endurance is godlike.
—HENRY WADSWORTH LONGFELLOW

Date: ____________________

TOPIC: *Are you as scared as I am? . . .*

Date:

TOPIC: *Please talk with me. I feel you're holding so much inside . . .*

Rather than love, than money, than fame,
give me truth.
—HENRY DAVID THOREAU

Date: ______

TOPIC: *I'm so thankful you're by my side . . .*

Date: ______________________________

TOPIC: *Sometimes I'm reluctant to let you know the pain (physical or emotional) I'm in . . .*

Date: ______

TOPIC: *It feels as if you want me to be the same as I was before the illness. You want me to be my good old self . . .*

All things are changed and we change with them.

—LOTHAIR I

Date: ___

TOPIC: *I feel you moving away from me . . .*

Date: ______________________

TOPIC: *I'm concerned your feelings for me will change . . .*

Date:

TOPIC: *What I'm learning from our relationship . . .*

Date:

TOPIC: *More than ever now, I need you to ask me how I am . . .*

Date: ____________________

TOPIC: *You play such an important part in my life because . . . (you teach me, you give me, you show me . . .)*

Date: ______________________

TOPIC: *At times I wish . . .*

Date:

TOPIC: *I don't want to be a burden . . .*

Date: ____________________

TOPIC: *I'm sorry we . . .*

Date:

TOPIC: *I'm so happy we . . .*

Date: ______

TOPIC: *I've been hiding lately—it's just what I need to do right now . . .*

Date: ______________________________

T O P I C : *As you know, I've been depressed lately, and I'm learning that depression and the treatment I'm receiving go hand in hand. Please hang in there with me . . .*

Date: ______________________

TOPIC: *I'm so proud of you . . .*

Date: ______

TOPIC: *My thoughts of you today . . .*

Date: ____________________

TOPIC: *There's something I've never told you that I want you to know . . .*

Seize this very minute. What you can do or dream,
you can begin it. Boldness has genius, power,
and magic in it.

—JOHANN WOLFGANG VON GOETHE

Date: ______________________________

TOPIC: *Sometimes my fears get in the way of my being close to you . . .*

Date: ________________________________

TOPIC: *Our partnership/marriage gives me so much strength . . .*

Date: ______________________________

TOPIC: *Thank you for taking the time to listen to me talk about . . .*

Date: ______________________________

TOPIC: *Keeping communication open between us is very important to me. If you're having difficulty talking with me, please write me a letter. I'm very open to receiving one . . .*

I have never found, in anything outside of the four walls of my study, an enjoyment equal to sitting at my writing desk with a clean page, a new theme, and a mind awake.

—WASHINGTON IRVING

Date:

TOPIC: *Sometimes I need to be alone . . .*

Date: __________

TOPIC: *Thank you . . .*

Date: ______________________

T O P I C : *Dreams . . . Thoughts . . . Poems . . .*

Date: ____________________

TOPIC: *Thank you . . .*

LOVEMAKING

- Since the diagnosis/illness, I've noticed a change in my sexual desires . . .
- Since the diagnosis/illness, my feelings about making love . . .
- I wonder if being close to me now is difficult for you, because when we make love . . .
- What I want you to know is sometimes I like to be touched and sometimes I don't . . .
- It's uncomfortable for me to talk with you about __________ (nudity, lovemaking, sex drive . . .), so I'm going to write you a letter . . .
- When I make love with you, I feel . . .
- If there's something you want me to know about our lovemaking but you can't say it, please write me a letter . . .
- Changes in my body make me feel . . .
- I'm afraid . . .
- I'd really like you to . . .
- I want . . .

Date:

TOPIC:

Date: ______

TOPIC: ______

Date:

TOPIC:

Date:

TOPIC:

Date:

TOPIC:

REFLECTIONS TO MY PARTNER/SPOUSE

My favorite memories of us together are:

- How we met . . .
- When I realized I loved you . . .
- Our wedding . . .
- Milestones . . .
- Celebrations . . .
- Vacations . . .
- Favorite memories of you/us . . .

Date:

TOPIC:

Date:

TOPIC:

Date:

TOPIC:

Date:

TOPIC:

Date:

TOPIC:

Letters to My Children

Date: ______

TOPIC: *The time I have to spend with you has changed, and I feel . . .*

Date: ____

TOPIC: *I'm angry that this illness impacts our lives as much as it does . . .*

Date:

TOPIC: *Today you did something really special for me . . .*

Date: ______________________________

TOPIC: *You are special to me because . . .*

Date: ______________________________

TOPIC: *I am grateful for what you show me . . .*

Date: ____

TOPIC: *I am grateful for what you teach me . . .*

Date:

TOPIC: *I am grateful for what you give me . . .*

No act of kindness, no matter how small,
is ever wasted.
—AESOP

Date: ______

TOPIC: *My prayer for you . . .*

Date: ______

TOPIC: *It seems to me that you're having difficulty talking to me. How about writing me a letter . . .*

I am all ears.

—ANTHONY TROLLOPE

Date: ______

TOPIC: *I know you are afraid . . .*

I WANT TO SHARE WITH YOU

- The importance of having a good relationship with yourself . . .
- What I believe about God . . .
- How I feel about religion . . .
- Games I like to play with you . . .
- The importance of friendships . . .
- When I visited a state, country, special place . . .
- How you can share your feelings . . .
- The importance of self-esteem . . .
- My feelings about marriage and choosing a partner . . .
- What I'd like to share with you about sex . . .
- My favorite songs, books . . .
- My favorite recipes . . .
- How I feel about death . . .
- What I want to share with you about finances . . .
- What I want to share with you about school and learning . . .
- My love for you . . .
- I want to share with you . . .
- Your medical history . . .

Date:

TOPIC:

Date:

TOPIC:

Date:

TOPIC:

Date:

TOPIC:

Date:

TOPIC:

REFLECTIONS TO MY CHILDREN

- My pregnancy . . .
- The day you were born . . .
- Your firsts . . . (walking, words, day at school, kiss, date, love . . .)
- Your birthdays . . .
- Trips with you . . .
- Camps you went to . . .
- When you learned to drive . . .
- Family celebrations . . .
- Family weddings . . .
- Holiday memories . . .
- Your friends . . .
- What you enjoyed . . .
- What we enjoyed together . . .
- You in your childhood . . .
- You in your teens . . .
- You in your adulthood . . .
- Special memories . . .

Date:

TOPIC:

Date:

TOPIC:

Date:

TOPIC:

Date:

TOPIC:

Date:

TOPIC:

Letters to My Relatives and Friends

Dear God, be with my family and friends. Bring peace to their troubled spirits. Enable them to know that their love gives me strength. Help me to express my gratitude and appreciation to them for all they have done and are continuing to do. Let them feel free to bring me their own joys and sorrows that I may continue to participate in their lives even as they share mine.

May this be a time of inner searching, that I may appreciate more fully the good and the beautiful in life and labor to bring these to the lives of others . . .

—From *Gates of Healing*

Date:

TOPIC: *I need to let you know that I am ill . . .*

Date: ______

TOPIC: *I'm so glad you're in my life . . .*

The only gift is a portion of thyself.
—RALPH WALDO EMERSON

Date: ______________________________

TOPIC: *I've felt disoriented since the diagnosis, so please excuse me for being out of touch . . .*

Date: ____________________

TOPIC: *I'm the one with the illness, yet it has had a tremendous impact on you. It seems that by being close to me you have a piece of it too . . .*

Date: ______________________

TOPIC: *Now that I have been sick awhile, your phone calls and visits are not as frequent. I am feeling . . . (sad, forgotten, left out . . .)*

Date:

TOPIC: *I feel as if I am on an emotional roller coaster . . .*

Date:

TOPIC: *Thank you for listening . . .*

A faithful friend is the medicine of life.
—ECCLESIASTICUS 6:16

Date: ______________________

TOPIC: *I am angry . . .*

Date: ______

TOPIC: *Writing letters helps me say things I'm not comfortable saying face to face . . .*

Date: ______

TOPIC: *I feel as if you think this illness is contagious . . .*

Date: ______

TOPIC: *Since the illness, I feel you relate differently to me . . .*

Date: __________

TOPIC: *I feel you moving away from me . . .*

Date: ______________________

TOPIC: *I've been hiding lately—it's just what I need to do right now . . .*

Date: ______________________________

TOPIC: *It means so much to me to have your support at this time in my life . . .*

Date: ______________________________

TOPIC: *As you know, I've been depressed lately, and I'm learning that depression and the treatment I'm receiving go hand in hand. Please hang in there with me . . .*

Date: ______________________________

TOPIC: *Telling you about ______________ is very helpful to me . . .*

Date: ______________________________

T O P I C : *I wish you could talk more with me about the illness . . .*

Date: ____

TOPIC: *I feel like a burden to you . . .*

Date: ______________________

TOPIC: *It's difficult for me to ask—and at this time I really need your care, support, concern . . .*

Date: ______________________________

TOPIC: *I wish you would join a support group because it seems you're having difficulty with my being sick . . .*

Date: ______

TOPIC: *It feels as if you want me to be the same as I was before the illness. You want me to be my good old self . . .*

Date: ______

TOPIC: *It's hard to talk with you about . . .*

Date: ______

TOPIC: *I had a setback in treatment . . .*

Date: ____

TOPIC: *Your support and care inspire me and make me feel good . . .*

Date:

TOPIC: *I'm so thankful for our friendship . . .*

Date: ______________________

TOPIC: *Spending time with you means so much to me . . .*

Date: ________________________________

TOPIC: *Thank you for taking such good care of me; however, I want you to go out with our friends, even make new ones, and have some fun . . .*

Date: ____________________

T O P I C : *Keeping communication open between us is very important to me. If you're having difficulty talking with me, please write me a letter. I'm very open to receiving one . . .*

Date: ______

TOPIC: *I love you . . .*

Date: ____________________

TOPIC: *I don't want to lose your friendship . . .*

Date: ____________________

TOPIC: *I need you to be there for me . . .*

Date:

TOPIC: *Thank you . . .*

Date: ______________________

TOPIC: *Thank you . . .*

Date:

TOPIC: *Thank you . . .*

REFLECTIONS TO MY RELATIVES AND FRIENDS

- Our history together . . .
- Conversations I remember . . .
- Special occasions we've spent together . . .
- We laughed so hard . . .
- Favorite memories . . .
- What I've learned from you . . .

Date:

TOPIC:

Date:

TOPIC:

Date: ______________________

TOPIC: ______________________

Date:

TOPIC:

Date:

TOPIC:

3

Sample Journal Entries and Letters

HOW TO USE THE SAMPLE JOURNAL ENTRIES AND LETTERS

Dear Friend,

Welcome to an extraordinary chapter of your journal.

One of the greatest privileges we have had in writing this book has been talking with women and men of all ages who have been challenged by illness. Many of them kept journals and wrote letters after being diagnosed and living with their illness. When we asked if they would share their writings with us, we were met with an enthusiastic "yes!" You see, our new friends wished they had had *A Journal for Healing* when they were diagnosed. So it is with the greatest compassion and love they have contributed their letters and journal entries to our book.

Their writings are here to guide you. They are also here to provide inspiration, encouragement, and company from fellow travelers who want you to know that you're not alone.

A special thank-you to everyone who allowed us to include their powerful writings in *A Journal for Healing*.

Cathy and Robin

Sample Journal Entries

Date: January 9, 1995

Topic: Why me? . . .

This thought keeps going through my head: "Why me?" It repeats itself over and over again. I just don't understand—I eat well, I exercise, I take care of myself. So why did I get breast cancer? They just call it the early stages, but that doesn't matter—it's still breast cancer and I have it. It's so hard to make this make sense. It's so hard to figure it out. Did I do something wrong? Did I cause this? Is it my fault? These questions also pop up as I wonder, "Why me?" Just a bunch of questions that don't and can't get answered. It's really the first time I can't answer the question "Why me?" in a way that makes sense. I'm so scared, I'm so confused. I feel like a spinning top . . . in search of the answer to "Why me?" Knowing full well I'll never get it. This makes no sense and nobody knows anyway.

Cathy

Date: November 1992

Topic: Back to the hospital . . .

Oh well . . . it's back to the hospital. One more surgery, hopefully the last one. It's so strange . . . I feel confident in my surgeon, comfortable with the people at the hospital, yet underneath it all is raw terror. Fear!! of the process and of the procedures. I just want it over and to never have to do this again.

Marilyn

Date: August 1, 1994

Topic: Since the diagnosis, my life feels out of control . . .

I remember the day as if it were yesterday. I'd been driving around for a while, not really going anywhere special. Thoughts, fears, worries were controlling my mind. You see, a couple of weeks ago I'd been given a diagnosis so serious that I can't remember the name. What I do remember is that no one could predict the outcome. I couldn't believe it. One moment I was going to the doctor for what I thought was a minor ailment and the next I didn't know whether I was going to live or die. I just never thought this would happen to me.

Lately I can't sleep or eat so well . . . I'm scared about my future and my family's . . . sometimes I even cry. I haven't done that for years. The world seems like it's spinning faster than I ever remember. The doctor wants me to start treatment right away. She says that time is wasting. Friends and family look so sad all the time, and me, I have this glazed look in my eyes.

That day I realized how out of control I felt. Driving was just my way of trying to outrun this darn diagnosis. Writing helps calm me down. Getting it out on paper relaxes me.

Ted

Date: November 22, 1994

Topic: Life is different since the diagnosis . . .

Life is different now. I'm different since the diagnosis and illness entered my life. I just had a cup of coffee. Now, I'm getting on in years and must have had over 10,000 cups of coffee but I'd swear this was the best cup of coffee I ever drank. I'd always been in such a hurry to get up and get the day going that I don't think I ever took the time to truly enjoy and appreciate just how wonderful a cup of coffee could be. It had just been a habit, part of my morning routine. Now I appreciate life, people, coffee and so much more. I'll tell you, one of the best things about this thing in my body is that it has slowed me down, slowed me down a lot.

Francine

Date: November 1994

Topic: Dreams . . . Thoughts . . . Poems . . .

HOW ABOUT YOU?

If you were told you had HIV,
How very brave do you think you'd be?

Would you continue living your life as before
Or would you take time, begin to explore?

Would you seek out meaning in a world gone awry
Or would you gather your loved ones to say good-bye?

Would you take the newest drugs to help keep you strong
Or would you live your life like a daring rock song?

Would you have hope when your friends have all died
Or would you curse at your g-d until you cried your eyes dried?

Would you look at your life through a rose-colored lens
Or would you feel trapped like Daniel in the lion's den?

Would you harness your strength to do a good deed each day
Or would you turn the other cheek and do nothing but play?

How would you live if you had HIV?
How very brave do you think you could be?

Would you feel helpless when there is no good news
Or would you hop in your car, radio blasting, and cruise?

Would you face your shadow that has followed you along
Or would you tremble and shake because you're just not that strong?

Would you socialize, maybe seek out a mate,
Or would you channel-surf and isolate?

How would you live if you had HIV?
How very brave do you think you could be?

I have HIV and I cannot subtract
A feeling that death will soon tap me on the back.

So I do what I can to keep this virus at bay
So it does not haunt me each and every day.

Danny Pepper

Date: December 23, 1991

Topic: Feelings about older cancer patients in the adult office I was in. I was the youngest patient . . .

How do you comfort someone who's about to die?
Who thinks they can only give up.
Sometimes I feel I'm so high on my horse,
that everything's so fine, no trouble.
Untouchable from the man . . .
Then I see another rider fallen from their horse,
I go back, but I can't help them up.
I reach down as far as I can. Then I see the man coming.
I want to say, "Get up, get back on your
horse, we can take the man, knock him down!"
But I am speechless, I am alone, riding on.
My horse is strong, most of the others are weak, old, dying.
And the man comes strong, hard, fast.
My horse carries me, but I am weak.

I wish I had strength, to turn, take the man.
Drop the hammer, knock him, hurt him,
give him pain, fear, make him cry for help, wish for death.
Knock him down so hard that the man
won't come back no more . . . but on he comes,
tirelessly, while I trust in my horse, but for how long?

Curtis Kosky

Date: November 1990

Topic: I've been wanting to write . . .

Just sitting down to write. I have a lot on my mind, but nothing really in particular. I figure if I just type away, it will come out . . . whatever that may be. It's about 11 P.M., November 19, 1990, and it's weird. It's raining right now. It's very pleasant and soothing. I enjoy listening to it. It helps me think. I don't really know why I'm writing. I just am. I like to write and people are always telling me to write, so I guess I figured now would be as good a time as any. I've been wanting to write. I figure, I have all this time on my hands, I might as well use it doing something I enjoy doing. I decided that I should write about all the shit I've been going through. I've been told that that would be a good thing to write. But I didn't just want to write another book about cancer. That would be boring and anybody could do it. So I figured I could write about the lighter side of cancer. I mean, let's face it. I've got some funny stories to tell about all this shit. Cancer really does have an amusing side to it . . .

Looking at where this is going now, I have a feeling that whatever this turns out to be will be a combination of the lighter side of cancer and part two of my thesis. Once again, I have no idea why I'm writing. I just am. There will be no perfection anywhere in here. My sentences will be choppy, my spelling will suck, my grammar might confuse you, my paragraphs might not go together, my damn sentences might not go together, and the entire paper or story or book or whatever this will be will be jumpy, with no plot, no structure, no direction, and no clue. I'm just going to write what I feel like writing and if it fits, great, if not, oh well. You'll figure it out. Just don't expect a beautifully written and flowing paper, because this ain't it. I'm just talking to myself and you're listening in and my mind doesn't always follow a pattern that people can understand. Just ask any of my friends. They'll tell you that I love to talk and I frequently make no sense at all. Because I start one thing and forget what my point is, or even if I had a point, and then I jump to something new and then I jump back and say the exact opposite of what I said two minutes before . . .

Spencer D. Presler

Date: November 1990

Topic: Time to tell my friends . . .

I had to tell some people who were just as eager to find out the truth as I was. I was planning on being strong. Telling people who asked but not letting it out. I sat myself down, proud of the fact that my emotions were very well bottled up inside. The bell rang and people began to walk by. Various friends saw that something was up. They sat with me but for the most part there was silence. At this point it was getting harder to hold it in. Then Jeanine walked by. She put her hand on my shoulder and there was something about the way she touched me and looked into my eyes. I lost it. I couldn't hold it back anymore. The tears came pouring out. The fear and the pain were all being released, right there, in the middle of my school. And I couldn't do anything about it. Most kids walked by, knowing that it was none of their business. My friends just stood or sat by me. Holding me. Shaking their heads. They didn't know the facts, but they knew enough.

The next day I decided I wanted to go to school. I knew that it would be my last chance. I had been going to Brentwood for six years and I wanted a final day. A day I could enjoy, but a happy good-bye day. A day where I could say farewell to a school that through good and bad had made me who I am. A school I am very glad I went to. It's a very small private school, grades seven through twelfth, with around 500 students. The small size had made my dad's death easier because the faculty and administration all knew me and my mom personally, so my situation was dealt with on a very personal basis. Also, because the student body is so small my entire class and much of the rest of the school gathered behind me and my mom in full support and gave us so much direct love and support that it really made things easier to deal with. So I had great feelings of love for Brentwood and I wanted to give it a proper so-long. I needless to say wasn't planning on going to school for scholastic reasons that day. So I showed up late and just kinda hung out in the quad. Various students came up to me and expressed their concern and well wishes. Many friends sat with me and to my surprise gave me gifts. All of which made me feel great. Some people may say that man is naturally evil. Fuck that. The people I was around that day showed me that humans are damn fine people and really care.

All day people offered massive love, support, concern, and general well wishes. I mean people I don't know and people I didn't know knew or gave a shit about me. Just everybody was great. And I was happy. Scared, but happy. I liked the attention, I loved the love, and it felt good. It was a positive day. Nobody was negative. No tears were shed. It was all smiles. I finished the day and said good-bye and got a bit sentimental and sad but kept my happiness nonetheless. It was just hard to say good-bye in one day to a school and to people I had spent the last six years growing up with. I went home. I can't remember what sort of mood I was in. I mean, I was happy and positive because it had been such a great day, but it was tough because I knew that from that moment on, my high school career was over and I was about to begin this horrible adventure. Within twenty-four hours I was going to be in the hospital, a place I had never been before. Within twenty-four hours I was going to be getting chemotherapy. Within twenty-four hours my life would go from one end to another. Within twenty-four hours my life would take a hiatus from teenage-hood and begin something your average teen wouldn't and shouldn't have to go through. All within twenty-four little hours.

Spencer D. Presler

Date: May 14, 1995

Topic: Mother's Day . . .

Today was Mother's Day and while I was not able to be with my mother, I was able to appreciate her presence in my life. She called me twice this week sounding concerned about me. I wanted her to know that I loved her and that she had given me one of the most important tools to deal with AIDS, strength. While I know that is not enough for her, I wanted to make sure I said it. The gift that AIDS has given me is the knowledge that I must say what I want to say and, more important, say it when I feel it. I was struck by the growth of my relationship with Robert's mother. I have two mothers now as well as two families. Despite feeling stressed about school and still reeling from bad lab reports from the doctor, I feel blessed. Blessed that my mother is such an important part of my life. Blessed that I have another mother that I share with Robert. And blessed that I had this day to do things I needed and wanted to do. I do have AIDS, but for now things are great. On some level I feel that nothing is going to happen to me right now. While I'm open to that changing, I trust that things will be right. I have never in my life felt as safe and secure in my life as I have these past few years. I don't think I would have a chance to feel this way if it were not for AIDS. For now, the good far outweighs the bad in my life.

Carlos

Date: April 10, 1995

Topic: My body—how it's changed . . .

Just when I'm feeling good about my life and breast cancer decisions, I look in the mirror and I realize I only have half a breast. I just sat down and cried. I wasn't prepared for this . . . I had no idea that the fact that my breast was the same size was due to swelling. I even remember them saying that . . . it just did not register. Being as obsessed as I am with my body, this is very difficult. Right now I don't know what to do or where to go . . . I feel lost, alone and unsure. I feel so devastated that this is how I'll look the rest of my life. I just can't believe it!

Cathy

Date: August 18, 1993

Topic: We went to a couples' support group . . .

Tonight was the first night we went to Ronnie Kaye's couples' workshop. It was very helpful for me. Tom also felt good about it. It's good for me to hear the partner's perspective and to hear other women struggle with their husband's wanting to make it all better. It helps me deal with the resentment I feel that Tom tries to make the cancer go away, that he just wants it gone and that there's really nothing he can do to take it away. He's doing what he can to listen to me and to support me in the way I ask. I just have to remember to ask (which I know is hard for me).

Heather

Date: December 18, 1991

Topic: My feelings around Christmas . . .

Sometimes I wonder why, just why, this all happened to me. I understand that it was random, that it just happened to be me, and I don't blame anyone else, or think someone or anyone deserves this instead of me. I just wonder why it had to happen, why did my life have to get so screwed up. Some things, only a few things, have made me happy—guitar, a few friends, writing, music, thinking of her—but mostly, everything has gone wrong and depressed me. It's not as much the fact that I have cancer, or the long treatments, or even losing my hair, but having to leave school, where I was finally being who I wanted to be and had made some good friends, people I really liked, and now having everybody have a different opinion. It is such a sudden change; I'm in such a spotlight. I really don't know if I can handle it. I would like to go somewhere new, fresh, to be an unknown and start over, where no one has any preconceived ideas about me. I can put on a face for any occasion, but when the clock strikes 12 midnight, will they still like who they see? Problem is, I don't know who he is either. I will look back someday and think it was nothing. Even now I sometimes forget, that is when I feel the best, those few minutes of normal living, but right now I am in the middle of it all. Hopefully, it goes by quickly, so I can get back on track, but until then, I hope I can survive.

Curtis Kosky

Date: April 29, 1995

Topic: Thank you . . .

I want to remember how thankful I feel much of the time these days. The most special people are:

Michael—for your enduring support, care, love and humor.

Katie—for your kindness, sensitivity and laughter.

Johnnie—for your concern and keeping me on my toes with your "Mom don't be in denial."

Mom—for going to the visits with me as much as you have.

Laurie—for being there so much, especially at the hospital.

Robin—for your beautiful friendship, going with me to so many visits, your incredible insights and gift of perception.

To many others, so many I can't have room for all of you . . . THANK YOU!!! for all the support you have given me.

Cathy

Date: January 10, 1995

Topic: People have been incredible . . .

Yesterday I was home and needed to call Clyde, the man who washes my car. He's such a nice guy. I already know that but when I told him I wouldn't be there on Friday because I had had surgery for breast cancer, he was incredible. Right there on the phone he began to pray. He asked me to join him in a prayer and he said the most sensitive and beautiful things as he prayed for "this demon cancer to be taken from her body." I cried from awe, disbelief and honor that he cared so much. It was truly amazing and felt so powerfully healing.

Cathy

Sample Letters

Date: May 11, 1995

Topic: To Family and Friends . . .

Dear Loved Ones,

I wanted to take a moment to tell you all how much you mean to me. My life is enriched by all of your presence. I can deal with anything so long as I have the unconditional love that we have all come to share. This illness may take my life, but so may driving on the Southern California freeways. Whatever the cause, I will go knowing that I loved and allowed myself to be loved. It will not matter whether I complete graduate school or not. I was allowed to share my life as well as be a part of some wonderful people's lives. I believe that the lesson of life is learning to love. Along with that goes learning to be loved and being vulnerable to hurt. I only have one hope. I hope that when the day comes that I pass out of your lives, that you take something from it. Everything happens for a reason. While it may not be evident immediately what the meaning of my presence in your lives is, it is there. Your presence in my life continually gives me love, hope and more lessons about my life. I will certainly have regrets, but I will only regret not seeing the culmination of all your lives. I want to see Jeremy and Stacee graduate from high school. Mom, I want to see you secure in your life. I hope to have a better history with my daughter Amy. And most important, I want to see Robert reach his personal goals. There are many other things I want to see and may not. But, half the fun of doing something is the ride there. The ride so far has been wonderful; whether or not I get there with you is irrelevant. All I will take with and all I leave behind me is the time and love shared with each and every one of you.

Carlos

Date: Sunday, June 3, 1994, 2 A.M.

Topic: Feelings about dying . . .

Dear Jake,

I've been tossing and turning in bed thinking about what you asked me today. Your question caught me by surprise and I got all tongue-tied. One moment we were busy with our jigsaw puzzle and the next moment you were asking me if I was scared of dying. I guess you could see how uncomfortable I was because you just patted my arm and said, "Never mind, Grandpa."

I'm sorry I couldn't answer you then. Death has always been such a private thing. No reason for it to be, that's just what I learned.

Jake, watching me live with this illness has been scary for you. I try not to talk about it when you're around. You're only eight and, well, I want to protect you from any worries you might have. I realized today, I can't do that anymore. What I can do is talk with you honestly and do my best to answer your questions.

Am I afraid of dying? A little. Not nearly as much as I used to be, however, and that's because of some very wonderful experiences I had a while back after your grandma Alice died. I never told anyone about this before and I want to tell you. It's brought me comfort. Maybe it will do the same for you.

It was a beautiful morning and I was missing Alice so much. I decided I'd work in the garden, do my best to keep it as lovely as she had. That morning I found the most beautiful peach rose. I carefully clipped it off and brought it in the house. I put it in Alice's favorite vase and placed it in our bedroom on her nightstand. As I stepped back to admire its beauty, I smiled. How she loved roses. I was peaceful in memories. It was then I felt someone was there, only I couldn't see them with my eyes. I sure could feel whoever it was. I sat on the edge of the bed still looking around. No one, just me and the breeze that ruffled the curtains as it traveled into our room.

While I was sitting there with this, well, invisible visitor, I remembered a story my neighbor Joe told me about some years back after his wife Beth Anne had died. He said one night he awoke with a jolt and felt he had company in his room. That's what he called it. Company. It was familiar company. He figured it was Beth Anne coming to say good night. He visited with her for a while, said good night, he told me, then went back to sleep. "Poor guy," I remember thinking. "The strain of her death has shook him up real bad, now he's having one of those hallucinations."

Was I having one of those hallucinations myself or was Alice visiting me? I looked around the room again. No one was there but me and my company. I took a big breath and began to relax a little. "Alice," I said, "is that you?"

My company and I sat together awhile longer. I was peaceful. The pain of missing Alice so much was easing up. I figured it must be Alice come to check up on me. I talked awhile. Told her what I'd been doing, making sure that the garden was looked after, that my cooking was getting better and that I missed her so much it hurt. I talked about a few more things I'd like to keep to myself. When I was finished, I thanked her for visiting me and asked her, if she could, to come back again. I felt Alice begin to leave. Now don't ask me how, I just did.

I stood up and stretched my legs. I know without a doubt that Alice had come back to check on me and let me know she was all right.

I've felt her company on many occasions since that morning, though not quite as often as I did after she died.

You see, Jake, those visits with your grandma let me know that we do go on. The word I hear my friends use is *spirit*—our spirits go on. After we die, we take on a different form, an invisible one. Death is just no longer a mystery for me.

I've thought about me dying a lot, Jake, and I'm not so scared anymore. I think more about how you and the family will do after I'm gone. So, after you read this letter please come and talk with me. If you have any questions, I promise I'll do my best to answer them. You can write me a letter, too, if talking feels awkward. (And don't mind your spelling, you know I don't care about that.)

Thanks, Jake, for asking me if I was scared of dying.

The sun's about to come up. I've been writing and thinking for a while now.

I love you.

Grandpa

Date: March 1995

Topic: Communication with my doctor . . .

Dear Dr. _________,

Upon picking up my X rays this morning, I found a copy of a letter you sent to my OB-GYN. At the bottom you mentioned I had canceled my appointment and would be "picking up my films and presumably taking them elsewhere for evaluation."

There are specific reasons why I canceled my appointment and took my films elsewhere. When I returned your phone call last week, you abruptly told me I had a lump in my breast and that I needed to come back in for further tests. When I began to ask questions such as which breast the lump was in and the size of the lump, you became very impatient, rude, and cold. You couldn't wait to pass me back to the front desk to make an appointment.

I just coauthored a book for individuals entitled *A Journal for Healing*. We specifically address the doctor/patient relationship and the importance of that relationship. Our phone conversation left me feeling scared, uninformed, and that you had no concern for me, the patient.

I was referred to Parkside Radiology Women's Center by my sister. The receptionist gave me more time than you or your staff did. She took her time, answered my questions, was compassionate and understanding, which left me feeling cared for—very important, I'm sure, to any woman who's just been told she has a lump in her breast.

The next time you speak with a woman to tell her she has a lump in her breast, I hope you will remember this letter and remember to consider the information you are giving her and the impact it will have. The results, contrary to my experience, can only be positive.

Robin F. Bernstein

PS: I informed my doctor of my decision to go elsewhere and he was very supportive. I also asked him to think twice before he refers his patients to your facility, regardless of your experience and expertise.

CLOSING LETTER FROM CATHY AND ROBIN

Dear Friend,

"Now that I have completed this journal, what can I do?" This might be the question you are asking yourself. We have a few suggestions. Go to your local bookstore and buy a blank journal or go to a stationery store and buy a three-ring notebook or a pad of paper. It can be quite simple. Its purpose is for you to have a source to continue the journal- and letter-writing process. If you wish, take topics from *A Journal for Healing* and place them inside your new journal or even begin anew. Design your new journal any way you wish.

Our hope is that you continue to write so you are able to understand what's going on within your world and what you can do about it.

We care very much about you. As you look back on the road you have traveled, at times there were unexpected detours taking you on a new path before returning you to the road on which you began. There have been storms forcing you to go inside. At times you have stopped off the road and had a picnic, played baseball, read a book, laughed and rested. Sometimes the fog prevented you from seeing what was ahead or even around you. There have also been times when the sky was bluer than you ever remembered and the sunshine warmed your soul. We don't know what the road ahead has in store, probably a little of what you have already seen and, for sure, surprises. It has been a privilege to be a part of this portion of your journey. We wish you wellness, always.

Love,

Cathy and Robin

ACKNOWLEDGMENTS

Thank you to everyone at Main Street Books who worked on *A Journal for Healing.* Special thanks to our editor, Lori Lipsky, and her assistant, Frances Jones.

Thank you to our agent, Susan Golomb. Throughout the ups and downs, you're always there for us.

Thank you to all the courageous people who spent time talking with us. Your experiences and insight enriched our lives and gave *A Journal for Healing* its essence.

Thank you to Michael and Nat—our husbands—whose kindness, support, and love helped us each step of the way.

Thank you to Katie, Johnnie, and Matthew—our children—whose spirit, enthusiasm, and joy of life brightens every day of our lives.

Love,

Cathy and Robin

SUGGESTED READING LIST/ BIBLIOGRAPHY

Ahn, Jung, M.D., and Ferguson, Gary. *Recovering from a Stroke.* New York: HarperCollins, 1992.

Ahronheim, Judith, M.D., and Weber, Doran. *Final Passages.* New York: Simon and Schuster, 1992.

Anderson, Gary. *Healing Wisdom.* New York: Dutton, 1994.

Ashe, Arthur. *Days of Grace.* New York: Ballantine Books, 1993.

Atwood, Glenna with Hunnewell, Lila. *Living Well with Parkinson's.* New York: John Wiley and Sons, 1991.

Brennan, Barbara Anne. *Hands of Light: A Guide to Healing Through the Human Energy Field.* New York: Bantam Books, 1988.

Brooks, Svevo. *The Art of Good Living: Simple Steps to Regaining Health and the Joy of Life.* Boston: Houghton Mifflin, 1990.

Broyard, Anatole. *Intoxicated by My Illness and Other Writings on Life and Death.* New York: Fawcett/Columbine, 1992.

Burnham, Sophy. *A Book of Angels.* New York: Ballantine Books, 1990.

Cederberg, Donna. *Breast Cancer? Let Me Check My Schedule!* Washington: Innovative Medical Education Consortium, 1994.

Chopra, Deepak, M.D. *Ageless Body, Timeless Mind.* New York: Harmony Books, 1993.

———. *Quantum Healing*. New York: Bantam Books, 1989.

Coughlin, Ruth. *Grieving: A Love Story*. New York: Random House, 1993.

Cousins, Norman, M.D. *Anatomy of an Illness as Perceived by the Patient*. New York: W. W. Norton, 1979.

Dackman, Linda. *Affirmations, Meditations, and Encouragements for Women Living with Breast Cancer*. Los Angeles: Lowell House, 1991.

Duff, Kat. *The Alchemy of Illness*. New York: Bell Tower, 1993.

Epstein, Gerald, M.D. *Healing Visualizations: Creating Health with Imagery*. New York: Bantam Books, 1989.

———. *Healing into Immortality*. New York: Bantam Books, 1994.

Fabien, Carol, M.D., and Warren, Andrea, M.A. *Recovering from Breast Cancer*. New York: HarperCollins, 1992.

Gendler, J. Ruth. *The Book of Qualities*. New York: Harper and Row, 1988.

Greenwood, Michael, M.D., and Nunn, Peter, M.D. *Paradox and Healing*. Canada: Paradox Publishers, 1992.

Hart, Judy. *Love, Judy: Letters of Hope and Healing for Women with Breast Cancer*. California: Conari Press, 1993.

Hirshaut, Yasher, M.D., and Pressman, Peter, M.D. *Breast Cancer: The Complete Guide.* New York: Bantam Books, 1992.

Huffington, Arianna. *The Fourth Instinct: The Call of the Soul.* New York: Simon and Schuster, 1994.

Jaffe, Hirshel, and Poller, H. Leonard, eds. *Gates of Healing.* New York: Central Conference of American Rabbis, 1988.

Kaye, Ronnie. *Spinning Straw into Gold: Your Emotional Recovery from Breast Cancer.* New York: Simon and Schuster, 1991.

Keay, Kathy. *Laughter, Silence, and Shouting: An Anthology of Women's Prayers.* San Francisco: Harper San Francisco, 1994.

Kubler-Ross, Elisabeth. *AIDS—The Ultimate Challenge.* New York: Macmillan, 1987.

———. *Living with Death and Dying.* New York: Macmillan, 1981.

———. *On Death and Dying.* New York: Macmillan, 1969.

———. *Working It Through.* New York: Macmillan, 1982.

Langone, John. *AIDS: The Facts.* Boston: Little, Brown, 1991.

LaTour, Kathy. *The Breast Cancer Companion.* New York: Avon Books, 1993.

LeShan, Lawrence. *Cancer as a Turning Point: A Handbook for People with Cancer, Their Families and Health Professionals.* New York: Plume, 1994.

Louden, Jennifer. *The Women's Comfort Book: A Self-Nurturing Guide for Restoring Balance in Your Life.* San Francisco: HarperCollins, 1992.

Lounsbury, Charles, and Darling, Harold. *Pictures in the Fire.* Washington: Blue Lantern Books, 1993.

Love, Susan, M.D. *Dr. Susan Love's Breast Book.* Massachusetts: Addison-Wesley, 1991.

Moore, Thomas. *Care of the Soul.* New York: HarperCollins, 1992.

Moyers, Bill. *Healing and the Mind.* New York: Doubleday, 1993.

Nixon, Daniel. *The Cancer Recovery Eating Plan.* New York: Random House, 1994.

Norris, Gunilla. *Sharing Silence: Meditation Practices and Mindful Living.* New York: Bell Tower, 1994.

Nuland, Sherwin B. *How We Die: Reflections on Life's Final Chapter.* New York: Knopf, 1994.

Passidomo-Trafford, Angela. *The Heroic Path: One Woman's Journey from Cancer to Self-Healing.* California: Hay House, 1993.

Pelletier, Kenneth. *Mind as Healer, Mind as Slayer.* New York: Dell, 1977.

Pinskey, Laura, and Douglas, Paul Harding, with Metroka, Craig. *The Essential HIV Treatment Book.* New York: Simon and Schuster, 1992.

Popham, Melinda Worth. *Skywater.* New York: Ballantine Books, 1990.

Progoff, Ira. *At a Journal Workshop: The Basic Text and Guide for Using the Intensive Journal Process.* New York: Dialog House Library, 1995.

Rainier, Tristine. *The New Diary.* Los Angeles: J. P. Tarcher, 1978.

Rhondell. *Headlines.* California: Rhondell Publishing Company (distributed by Harmony Workshop, Inc., a nonprofit educational foundation), 1993.

———. *Notes on Personal Integration and Health.* California: Rhondell Publishing Company, 1993.

Rollin, Betty. *First, You Cry.* New York: HarperCollins, 1976.

Rossman, Martin, M.D. *Healing Yourself: A Step-by-Step Program for Better Health Through Imagery.* New York: Simon and Schuster, 1987.

Satir, Virginia, Ph.D. *Self-Esteem.* California: Celestial Arts, 1975.

Sherline, Reid. *Love Anyhow: Famous Fathers Write to Their Children.* New York: Timken, 1994.

Siegel, Bernie, M.D. *Love, Medicine and Miracles.* New York: HarperCollins, 1986.

———. *Peace, Love and Healing.* New York: Harper and Row, 1989.

Simonton, Carl, M.D., and Henson, Reid, with Hampton, Brenda. *The Healing Journey.* New York: Bantam Books, 1992.

Simonton, Carl, M.D., Mathews-Simonton, Stephanie, and Creighton, Joseph. *Getting Well Again*. New York: Bantam Books, 1992.

Soffa, Virginia. *The Journey Beyond Breast Cancer.* Vermont: Healing Arts Press, 1994.

Stoddard, Alexandra. *Gift of a Letter.* New York: Doubleday, 1990.

———. *Making Choices: The Joy of a Courageous Life.* New York: Morrow, 1994.

Swirsky, Joan, and Balaban, Barbara. *The Breast Cancer Handbook.* New York: HarperCollins, 1994.

Veary, Nana. *Change We Must: My Spiritual Journey.* Hawaii: Water Margin Press, 1989.

About the Authors

Cathy Moore, Ph.D., is a licensed clinical psychologist. She lives in Redondo Beach, California, with her husband, Michael, and two children, Katie and Johnnie. Robin Freeman Bernstein, M.A., is a licensed Marriage Family Child Therapist. She lives in Santa Monica with her husband, Nat, and son, Matthew.

Through years of private practice, and in a number of ventures as partners, the authors have helped guide hundreds of clients—children, adolescents, adults, couples, and families—to better understand themselves and maximize their full potential.

The authors are currently working on a series of journals focusing on the different stages of life. The first of these, *Letters for Tomorrow: A Journal for Expectant Moms and Dads*, was published by Doubleday in February 1995.

Dear Friends.

We are beginning a new book entitled *Letters of Courage and Hope for Those Challenged by Illness*. It will be a collection of letters, journal entries, poems, inspirational stories, and words of wisdom that will give the reader inner strength and the knowledge that they are not alone. If you have a story of hope or a message to share with others we would be honored to include it in this book. Please write to us:

Cathy Moore and Robin Freeman Bernstein
253A 26th Street, Suite 178
Santa Monica, CA 90402

Please be aware that by writing to us, you are giving permission to be quoted in the book. Thank you for your contribution.

With Appreciation,

Cathy and Robin